The Trending Diabetes Preparations

Explore the Innovations on Diabetes Diet through the Current Trends

By

Tiara Crocker

TABLE OF CONTENTS

INTRODUCTION 8

CHAPTER 1 BREAKFAST RECIPES 10

1.1 Beans and Microwave-Poached Egg.................. 11

1.2 Oatmeal Smoothie 14

1.3 Mushroom and Spring Onion Omelet 15

1.4 Breakfast Sandwich 17

1.5 Almond Flour Banana Bread............................19

CHAPTER 2 SNACKS 22

2.1 Blueberry Smoothie... 23

2.2 $^1/_3$ Cup Edamame... 24

2.3 ¾ Cup Frozen Mango Cubes 25

2.4 Yogurt with Sunflower Seeds.......................... 26

2.5 No fat Greek Yogurt with Honey 27

2.6 Baked Potato and Salsa................................... 28

2.7 Pistachios 29

2.8 One Cup Grapes 30

CHAPTER 3 SALADS RECIPES....................31

3.1 Healthy Apple and Curried Chicken Salad 32

3.2 Arugula Salad with Lemon Vinaigrette Dressing with steak 34

3.3 Fattish Salad...37

3.4 Lemon Pea Salad.. 39

3.5 Calico Slaw 40

3.6 Grill Corn Salad.. 42

CHAPTER 4 SOUPS & STEWS 44

4.1 Leek & butter bean soup with crispy kale & bacon 45

4.2 Spiced lentil & butternut squash soup 47

4.3 Winter vegetable & lentil soup 49

4.4 Chickpea tagine soup 51

4.5 Cauliflower soup 53

4.6 Herby broccoli & pea soup..............................55

CHAPTER 5 POULTRY 57

5.1 Zippy Turkey Zoodles 58

5.2 General Cho's Stew 60

5.3 Perfect Roast Chicken 62

5.4 Baked Turkey with Onions & Leeks................. 65

5.5 Cheesy Chicken and Broccoli 67

CHAPTER 6 FISH AND SEAFOOD 69

6.1 Salmon Alfredo... 70

6.2 One-Pot Pasta with Tuna.................................72

6.3 Greek Tuna Casserole 74

6.4 Easy Thai Green Curry with Shrimp 77

6.5 Grilled Shrimp Skewer with Creamy Chili Sauce
....79

CHAPTER 7 VEGETABLES RECIPES 81

7.1 Stir-Fry Rice Bowls... 82

7.2 Spinach Quesadillas 84

7.3 Quick Mushroom Barley Soup......................... 86

7.4 Hummus & Veggie Wrap-Up 88

7.5 Zucchini Crust Pizza.. 90

CHAPTER 8 PORK LAMB & BEEF 92

8.1 Succotash Salad with Grilled Sirloin................ 93

8.2 Stir-Fried Green Beans with Steak & Peanuts 96

8.3 Pressure Cooker "Corned" Beef & Cabbage..... 98

8.4 Lamb Chops with Orange Sauce.................... 100

8.5 Marinated Leg of Lamb 102

CHAPTER 9 DESSERTS.............................104

9.1 Peanut Butter Swirl Chocolate Brownies........105

9.2 No-Bake Coconut Cream Pie 108

9.3 Creamy Strawberry-Banana Tart................... 110

9.4 Raspberry Crumble Bars............................... 113

9.5 Low Carbs Chocolate mug cake with Coconut Flour... 117

CONCLUSION 119

INTRODUCTION

There are tons of methods for improving your nutrition but it is only a way to do it properly. With this book you are going to experience a new scenario of choices that includes low carbs, grains, delicious sauces and amazing tips for take good care of your Diabetic Condition.

It is important to clarify that this diet is a lifestyle that not only make your body feel better, also helps the brain and the rest of important organs to detox. Did you ever ask yourself if there is a way to improve your routine? Or maybe something that makes you feel proud of yourself? If that is your case, this book is a hidden treasure that you must have!

We will include easy recipes that you can do whenever you want and quick advices to follow this great preparations like:

1. - Grains & Beans in an innovated way.

2. - Awesome sauces for all occasions.

3. - Variety of fun breakfast.

This diet is often mistaken with vegan or vegetarian diets for similar reasons. However, these diets are not the same, but in some respects, they are related.

CHAPTER 1 BREAKFAST RECIPES

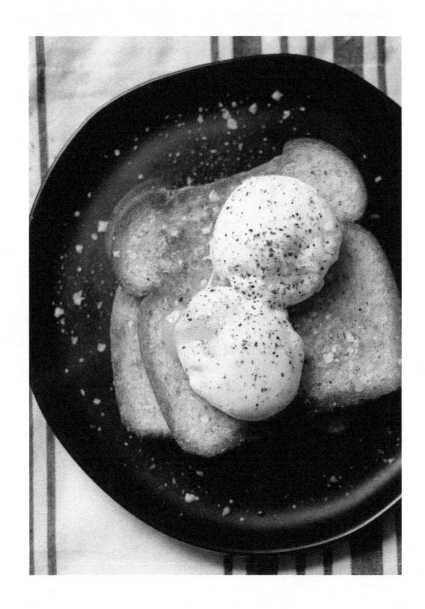

1.1 Beans and Microwave-Poached Egg

This recipe is called by Gallo pinto in Costa Rica, it means a spotted rooster, because of the dark beans on the white rice.

(**Prep. time:** 15 min. | **Servings:** 2 | **Difficulty:** medium)

Serving size: ¾ cup bean mixture + 1 egg + 1 tbsp. cheese + ¼ avocado

Per serving: Kcal 364, Fat 20g, Net Carbs 32g, Proteins 17g

Ingredients

- ¼ cup red bell pepper, chopped
- 2 tsp. canola oil
- 2 scallions, chopped, greens and whites separated
- ¾ cup canned black beans, low sodium, rinsed
- ½ tsp. ground cumin
- ½ cup of barley, cooked
- ⅛ tsp. salt
- ½ cup chicken or vegetable broth, cooked
- ⅛ tsp. hot sauce
- 2 large eggs
- 1 cup water
- 1 tsp. distilled white vinegar
- ½ sliced avocado
- 2 tbsp. pepper Jack cheese, shredded
- 2 tbsp. fresh cilantro, coarsely chopped

Directions

1. Add oil in a pan and heat it on medium heat. Add scallion whites, cumin, and bell pepper; cook, stirring frequently, until soft, for about 1-2 min. Add beans, broth, salt, and cooked barley. Cook until the majority of the liquid in the pan is absorbed, about 3-5 minutes. Add hot sauce and scallion greens, stir. Transfer the contents equally into 2 bowls.

2. Add half teaspoon vinegar and half cup water in a microwave-safe bowl. Crack an egg into the bowl and make sure the egg submerged completely. Cover the bowl with a plate and microwave it on high for 1 minute till the egg yolk is still a little runny and the white is settled. Remove the poached egg with a spoon, pat it dry and place it on top of the bean mixture in 1 of the bowls. Repeat these steps to make another poached egg and also use it to top the beans.

3. Top the bowls with 1 tablespoon cheese and a quarter avocado, each. Garnish with cilantro.

Tips

To prepare ahead: Make barley and beans (Step 1) up to 2 days before and store in the fridge. Heat it in the microwave when desired and then go on to the second step

1.2 Oatmeal Smoothie

(**Prep. time:** 5min. | **Servings:** 2 | **Difficulty:** easy)

Per serving: Kcal 135, Fat 0g, Net Carbs 20g, Proteins 12g

Ingredients

- 1 cup uncooked oats

- 3 cups skimmed milk

- 2 frozen bananas, sliced into little chunks

- Sugar substitute (stevia or others)

- 2 tbsps. grounded flax-seed

- 2 tbsps. coffee extract

Directions

1. Ground the oats in a food processor.

2. Combine all the ingredients in a blender and blend.

1.3 Mushroom and Spring Onion Omelet

(**Prep. time:** 15 min. | **Servings:** 2 | **Difficulty:** easy)

Serving size: 50g

Per serving: Kcal 250, Fat 16.5g, Net Carbs 3g, Proteins 22g

Ingredients

- 2 eggs

- 1 tbsp. rapeseed oil

- A pinch of white pepper

- 150g sliced mushrooms

- 10g low-fat grated cheddar

- 1 chopped spring onion

Directions

1. Add the eggs and pepper in a bowl, beat and set aside.

2. Take a pan and heat the oil. Add spring onion and mushroom, and cook over medium heat for 5 minutes, until soft, stir regularly.

3. Mix and stir the eggs and mushroom mix then cook for 3 minutes, gently.

4. Transfer the omelet to a plate, sprinkle cheese on top, and fold it in half.

1.4 Breakfast Sandwich

(**Prep. time:** 1 hr. 10 min. | **Servings:** 12 | **Difficulty:** medium-hard)

Serving size: 1 sandwich

Per serving: Kcal 290, Fat 13g, Net Carbs 35g, Proteins 20g

Ingredients

- 12 large eggs

- 1 large chopped onion

- 4 cooked and diced chicken sausages

- 1 finely chopped bell pepper

- 5 big kale leaves, chopped and with ribs removed or baby spinach

- 1 tbsp. olive oil

- 1 tbsp. baking powder

- ¼ cup water or milk

- 12 thin burger buns, bagels, or English muffins (whole-wheat)

- 12 slices real cheese

- Cooking spray

- Salt

Directions

1. Preheat a large non-stick pan on medium heat and add oil. Add onions and fry for 3 minutes. Add the bell pepper and fry for 3 further minutes. Add kale, along with a pinch of pepper and salt; fry for one more minute. Stir regularly while frying.

2. Preheat your oven to 375°F and spray a large 11 x 16 baking sheet with your cooking spray. Add eggs, baking powder, milk, salt, and pepper, in a bowl; and whisk firmly. Add the cooked vegetables along with the sausage; and stir. Pour the mixture onto the baking sheet, distribute the sausages and vegetables evenly using a fork. Bake it uncovered, for 25 minutes.

3. Take out the eggs. Loosen the eggs from the edges with a spatula. Then cut the eggs into 12 equal parts.

4. Take 12 pieces of parchment and aluminum foil. Place the egg on the bottom bun and top with cheese. Close the bun. Wrap it in parchment paper and then in aluminum tightly.

Note:

Store in the fridge for up to 5 days or freeze in a bag for up to 3 months.

1.5 Almond Flour Banana Bread

(**Prep. time:** 1 hr. | **Servings:** 10 |**Difficulty:** medium)

Serving size: 1 slice

Per serving: Kcal 345, Fat 25g, Net Carbs 22g, Proteins 10g

Ingredients

- ¼ cup your desired sweetener
- 3 large eggs
- ¼ cup melted butter (or a mild oil)
- 1 tbsp. cinnamon
- 1 tbsp. vanilla extract liquid
- 1 tbsp. baking soda
- 3 large ripened bananas with brown spots
- ¼ tbsp. salt
- 1 tbsp. baking powder
- 3 cups almond flour

Directions

1. Preheat your oven to 350ºF, line a metal 5x9 loaf pan with paper parchment. Use cooking spray on just the bottom and the lower 1 inch. Set it aside.

2. Mash the bananas in a big mixing bowl. Add eggs, oil, vanilla, sweetener, cinnamon, baking powder, baking soda, and salt; mix them with a whisk until they are combined. Then add the almond flour and combine it by mixing with a spatula.

3. Pour the batter into the loaf pan and let it bake for about 50 min. Use a toothpick to confirm it is ready. Take it out from the oven, then let the bread cool for 10 min. Remove the bread from the loaf pan, let it cool for another 10 min. Slice and serve.

Note:

This bread can be stored in an airtight container or bag for up to 3 days.

CHAPTER 2 SNACKS

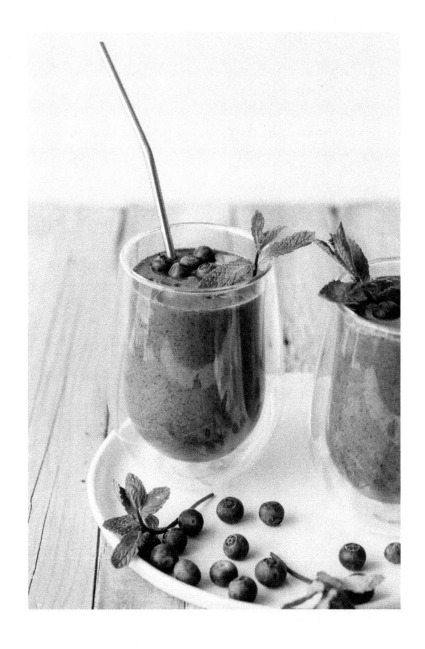

2.1 Blueberry Smoothie

A refreshing smoothie is a delicious way through the day to bring in some additional antioxidants and calcium. Aim to mix $^2/_3$ cup frozen blueberries with $^1/_3$ cup nonfat yogurt and ice. It's icy and refreshing. That slows you down in your ability to drink it speedily. Snacks that take longer to eat are also more rewarding.

2.2 ⅓ Cup Edamame

The healthiest snacks you can find in an aisle are these young soybeans. A half-cup provides about 8 g of Proteins and 4 g of fiber to help keep you healthy. You can get about 10 percent of your average regular iron quota as a bonus. For a fast snack on the go, Edamame is also available in ready-to-eat containers.

2.3 ¾ Cup Frozen Mango Cubes

You can purchase or produce these pre-packaged items yourself. It's like having frozen candy dessert. It's a great way to get fiber and beta-carotene while satisfying your sweet cravings. A ¾ cup portion contains only 90 calories and offers 60 percent of the prescribed daily vitamin C intake.

2.4 Yogurt with Sunflower Seeds

Mix a teaspoon of the sunflower seeds in half a cup of 0% fat yogurt. Seeds give a ton of texture, in just 19 calories. Yogurt is always a decent Proteins source, and the whole snack contains less than half a gram of fat. It's important to use sunflower seeds that are not salted, particularly if you're reducing your sodium intake.

2.5 No fat Greek Yogurt with Honey

Greek yogurt is renowned for its super fluffy texture and high Proteins quality. Only ½ cup of regular Greek yogurt provides 12 g of Proteins to keep you stay full. Pour on a teaspoon of honey, and it will add up to 84 calories to the entire snack. The best part of it is, you may sound like you're consuming dessert.

2.6 Baked Potato and Salsa

Microwaving a boiled potato for a simple snack filled with Vit. C and not calories. A half of medium baked potato produces 80 calories – hold the skin filled with nutrients. Place a tbsp. salsa on top the potato to mix it up and keep it below 100 calories.

2.7 Pistachios

Do not let your pistachios intake be intimidated by the high-fat content — most of it is unsaturated or "good" fat. Take 20 pistachios, and get in just 80 calories and less than one gram of saturated fat. Moreover, they are high in calcium, fiber, and other essential vitamin. and minerals. To stop an excessive dosage of sodium, consume them roasted raw or dry with no salt.

2.8 One Cup Grapes

Grapes are saturated with water, which ensures 100 calories in a full cup. The water content tends to give you a sense of fullness and leaves you hydrated. Grapes are also a good source of manganese and vitamin K and also provide some fiber. They are perfect consumed fresh or frozen.

CHAPTER 3 SALADS RECIPES

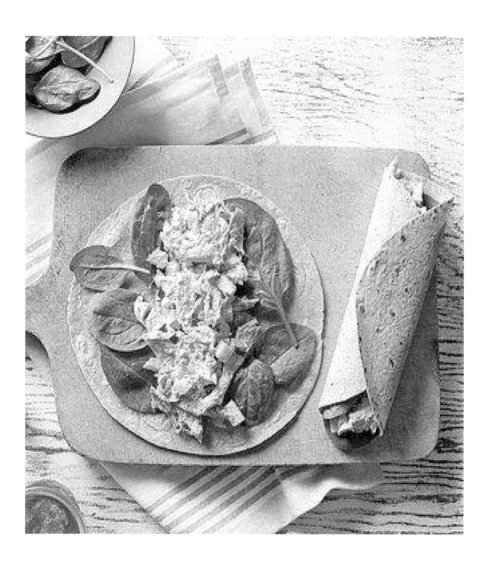

3.1 Healthy Apple and Curried Chicken Salad

This Balanced Apples and Curry Chicken Salad transforms a few easy substitutes into something delicious and nice for you to turn a traditionally unwholesome meal into full of nutrition!

(Prep. time: 10 min. | **Servings:** 5 | **Difficulty:** medium)

Serving size: 1/5th of recipe

Per serving: Kcal: 236, Fats: 5.6, Carbs: 8.5g Proteins: 28.9g

Ingredients

- 1 lb. chicken breast cooked, diced
- 1 diced Granny Smith apple
- 2 diced celery stalks
- 2 green onions
- ½ cup chopped cashews
- 1 cup regular, non- fat, Greek yogurt
- 1 tbsp. Tahini
- 4 tsp. curry powder

- 1 tsp. ground cinnamon

Directions

1. In a large mixing cup, add the tahini, yogurt, cinnamon, and curry powder.

2. Include celery, chicken, tomato, green onions, and cashews. Mix to blend. Salad can be eaten individually, as a sandwich, or with a papaya scooped out to give it more of an exotic feel.

Recipe Notes

1. This gives five portions of apple and chicken salad. You would need chicken breasts, which you can cook just before putting the salad together or 1 or 2 days.

2. When combined, the salad will remain fresh in the refrigerator for four days.

3.2 Arugula Salad with Lemon Vinaigrette

Dressing with steak

No wonder people with diabetes need to combine Proteins with Carbs to avoid increases in blood sugar. Having the Proteins from a finely cut steak makes your mouth water just dreaming about it. New tossed arugula, steak-toped, and served with a balsamic drizzle is perfect for the entire family!

(Prep. time: 20 min. | **Servings:** 4 to 6 | **Difficulty:** hard)

Serving size: 1 steak

Kcal: 357, Fats4.5g: Carbs: 31g, Proteins: 29g

Ingredients

- 1 lb. Thinly sliced London Broil

- ¼ cup lemon juice

- 6 cups arugula lettuce

- 2 tbsp. olive oil

- $1/3$ cup sliced red onion

- 1 tbsp. honey mustard

- 1 sliced green bell pepper

- 1 tsp. lemon zest

- ¼ tsp. salt and pepper

- ½ cup grated parmesan cheese

Directions

1. Toss onion arugula and bell pepper. Put a salad bowl on each platter.

2. Put a couple of slices of steak on each salad.

3. Mix ingredients for the seasoning together in a medium dish.

4. Drizzle the salad

3.3 Fattish Salad

Fresh Red cabbage gives this fattoush an extra crunch!

(**Prep. time:** 25 min. | **Servings:** 8 | **Difficulty:** easy)

Serving Size: 1 ½ cups

Per serving: Kcal: 109, Fats: 5.8, Carbs: 6g Proteins: 3g

Ingredient

- 2 whole-wheat pita bread, split and cut into 1-inch pieces
- ¼ cup lemon juice
- 2 tsp. extra-virgin olive oil
- ½ tsp. kosher salt
- ½ tsp. ground pepper
- 3 cups red cabbage, thinly sliced
- 3 cups Romaine lettuce, chopped
- 1 cup grape/cherry tomatoes, halved
- 2 sliced Persian cucumbers
- 2 scallions, thinly sliced
- 1 cup fresh parsley, chopped

Directions

1. Heat oven to 375°F.

2. Arrange cut up pita pieces in one layer on a large baking sheet. Bake, flipping once, until crispy, about 10 to 15 minutes. Let cool, about 5 minutes or until at room temperature.

3. In the meantime, mix oil, lemon juice, pepper, and salt in a large bowl. Add lettuce, tomatoes, cabbage, scallions, cucumbers, and parsley and toss. Add in the pita chips and toss until well combined.

3.4 Lemon Pea Salad

A favorite salad for a hot summer day.

(**Prep. time:** 10 min. | **Servings:** 1 | **Difficulty:** easy)

Serving size: 1 cup

Per serving: Kcal: 48, Fats: 0.6, Carbs: 9g Proteins: 3g

Ingredients

- 1 cup raw peas
- ½ lemon juiced
- Salt and ground black pepper, to taste

Directions

1. Mix all ingredients together in a bowl.
2. Serve.

3.5 Calico Slaw

Crunchy cabbage slaw with apples, peppers, and carrots.

(**Prep. time:** 50 min. | **Servings:** 8 | **Difficulty:** medium)

Serving size: 1/5th of recipe

Per serving: Kcal: 80, Fats: 0.3, Carbs: 19g Proteins: 2g

Ingredients

- 1 ½ head green cabbage, shredded

- 3 carrots, shredded

- 1 bell pepper green, seeded and thin slices

- 1 bell pepper red, seeded and thin slices

- 1 bell pepper yellow, seeded and thin slices

- 1 red delicious apple, cored and chopped

- 1 golden delicious apple, cored and chopped

- 2 tbsp. apple cider vinegar

- 2 tbsp. sugar substitute (Stevia or Splenda)

- ½ tsp. fine sea salt

- Ground black pepper, to taste

Directions

1. Toss the carrots, cabbage, red bell pepper, green bell pepper, and all apples together in a large bowl.

2. Mix the apple cider vinegar, sea salt and the sugar substitute together in a small bowl; add black pepper to taste. Pour the vinegar mixture on the cabbage mixture and toss gently to coat. Cover the bowl with plastic wrap and refrigerate for at least 30 minutes.

3.6 Grill Corn Salad

An easy and yummy side dish for hot summery days! Tastes excellent with your grilled lunches or to munch alone.

(**Prep. time:** 1hr 10 min. | **Servings:** 6 | **Difficulty:** medium)

Serving size: 1/6th of recipe

Per serving: Kcal: 103, Fats: 3, Carbs: 19g Proteins: 3g

Ingredients

- 6 ears farm fresh corn

- 1 green pepper, diced

- 2 ½ tomatoes, diced

- ¼ cup red onion, diced

- ½ bunch fresh cilantro, chopped or more

- 2 teaspoons or more olive oil

- Ground black pepper and salt, according to taste

Directions

1. Heat a grill to medium heat and slightly oil the grill.

2. Grill the corn until the corn is cooked and tender, turning occasionally and of black specks appear, for about 10 minutes; put aside until adequately cool to handle. Shred off the kernels and place in a bowl.

3. Mix the corn kernels while warm with the diced tomato, green pepper, cilantro, onion, olive oil. Sprinkle with pepper and salt; toss until mixed evenly. Put aside for at least 20 minutes to let flavors to merge beef.

CHAPTER 4 SOUPS & STEWS

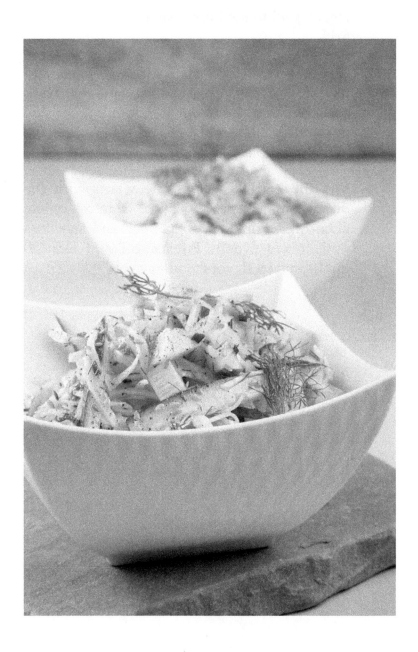

4.1 Leek & butter bean soup with crispy kale & bacon

(**Prep. time:** 30 min. | **Servings:** 4 | **Difficulty:** easy)

Serving size: 1 cup

Per serving: Kcal 274, Fat 12g, Carbs 21g, Proteins 14g

Ingredients

- 4 tsp. olive oil
- Sliced leek 500g
- 4 leaves picked thyme sprigs
- 2 cans butter beans of 400g
- Vegetable bouillon stock 500ml
- 2 tsp. wholegrain mustard
- ½ pack flat-leaf parsley
- 3 ashers streaky bacon
- Chopped kale 40g
- Chopped hazelnuts 25g

Directions

1. Heat 1 tablespoon of oil over low heat in a wide saucepan.

2. Add the leeks, thyme & season. Cover and cook until softened for 15 min., adding a splash of water as the leeks tend to stick.

3. Add butter beans with water from cans, stock and mustard. Bring to boil and cook until hot for 3-4 min.

4. Mix soup in food processor or a stick blender, mix in the parsley and stir for seasoning.

5. Place the bacon over medium heat into a big, non-stick frying pan. Cook until crispy for 3-4 minutes, then set aside to cool.

6. In the pan, add the resulting 1 tsp. oil, and tip into the kale & hazelnuts. Cook for 2 minutes, stirring till the kale is wilted and crisping at edges and hazelnuts are toasted. Cut the bacon into tiny pieces, then stir into the kale mixture.

7. Heat the soup and add a splash of water if it's too thick.

8. Serve in bowls filled with a combination of bacon & kale.

4.2 Spiced lentil & butternut squash soup

(**Prep. time:** 40 min. | **Servings:** 4-6 | **Difficulty:** easy)

Serving size: 1 cup

Per serving: Kcal 167, Fat 5g, Carbs 23g, Proteins 6g

Ingredients

- 2 tbsp. olive oil

- 2 onions finely chopped

- 2 garlic cloves, crushed

- ¼ tsp. hot chili powder

- 1 tbsp. ras el hanout

- Peeled & cut into 2cm pieces 1 butternut squash

- Red lentils 100g

- 1lb. hot vegetable stock

- Chopped coriander 1 small bunch + extra to serve

- Dukkah & natural yogurt to serve

Directions

1. Heat the oil over moderate to high heat in a broad flame-proof casserole platter or saucepan. Fry the onions for 7 minutes with a pinch of salt or until smooth and caramel-like. Add the garlic, chili and ras el hanout, and proceed to cook for 1 min.

2. Whisk in lentils and squash. Pour over the stock and to taste, season. Bring to simmer, then minimize heat to simmer & cook, covered, for 25 minutes or until soft. Blitz the soup until creamy with a stick blender, then season to taste. To freeze, leave to cool fully, then move to large freezer-proof containers.

3. Mix the coriander leaves and ladle the broth into bowls. Serve with dukkah, yogurt, and extra leaves of coriander on top.

4.3 Winter vegetable & lentil soup

(**Prep. time:** 30 min. | **Servings:** 2 | **Difficulty:** easy)

Serving size: 1 cup

Per serving: Kcal 264, Fat 3g, Carbs 37g, Proteins 16g

Ingredients

- Dried red lentils 85g

- 2 carrots quartered lengthwise then diced

- 3 sliced celery sticks

- 2 sliced small leeks

- 2 tbsp. tomato purée

- 1 tbsp. fresh thyme leaves

- 3 garlic cloves, chopped

- 1 tbsp. vegetable bouillon powder

- 1 tsp. ground coriander

Directions

1. Placed all the ingredients into a big saucepan. Spill over 1 and ½ liters of boiling water and mix well.

2. Cover & let cook for 30 minutes until the lentils and vegetables are tender.

3. Ladle in bowls & eat right away or blitz a third of the soup with a hand blender or with a food processor if you want a very thick texture.

4.4 Chickpea tagine soup

(**Prep. time:** 30 min. | **Servings:** 4 | **Difficulty:** easy)

Serving size: 1 cup

Per serving: Kcal 309, Fat 10g, Carbs 34g, Proteins 13g

Ingredients

- 2 red peppers
- 1 tbsp. rapeseed oil
- 1 red onion, thinly sliced
- 2 crushed garlic cloves
- 2 coriander, grounded
- 1 tsp. cumin, grounded
- Rose harissa paste 2 tbsp.
- 2 cans of chickpeas of 400g, drained and rinsed
- 1 ½ lb. low-salt veg stock
- Chopped kale 150g
- 1 lemon, zested and juiced
- Finely chopped dried apricot 50g
- ½ bunch finely chopped parsley

- Fat-free natural yogurt to serve optional

Directions

1. Heat the grill up to its maximum setting. Cut the peppers in half and deseed, then lay cut-side down on a foil-lined baking sheet. Grill for 10-15 minutes, or until softened & blistered. Leave until cold enough to handle, then cut the skins and dump them. Slice the roasted peppers into small strips.

2. Heat up the oil over low heat in a large saucepan. Fry the onion until softened for 8-10 min. Stir in the paste of harissa, garlic, coriander, and cumin, and simmer for a further 1 min. Put in the chickpeas and stock, bring to boil and cook for 15 minutes, sealed.

3. Mix the peppers through soup with the kale, the lemon zest and the juice and apricots and cook for another 5 minutes, sealed. Ladle the soup in bowls and serve with sprinkled diced parsley and a dollop of yogurt, if you prefer.

4.5 Cauliflower soup

(**Prep. time:** 25 min. | **Servings:** 4-6 | **Difficulty:** easy)

Serving size: 1 cup

Per serving: Kcal 176, Fat 8g, Carbs 14g, Proteins 8g

Ingredients

- 1 cauliflower, cut into florets
- ½ tbsp. ground cumin
- 2 tbsp. olive oil + extra for drizzling
- 4 thyme sprigs
- 1 chopped onion
- 1 chopped celery stick
- 1 crushed garlic clove
- Veg or chicken stock 750-850ml
- Single cream 100ml
- ½ bunch parsley, chopped

Directions

1. Heat the oven to 220°C.

2. Add 1 tbsp. of olive oil, cumin, and thyme to cauliflower florets in a roasting pan. Roast for 15 minutes or till soft, and golden. Discard thyme.

3. Heat the remaining oil with the onion and celery in a saucepan and fry at medium heat for 10 minutes or until softened. Stir in the garlic & cook 1 min. Stir in much of the cauliflower, reserving plenty to later top the soup. Add 750 ml of stock to the saucepan and simmer. Cook 10 minutes.

4. Blitz the soup using a hand blender/food processor until smooth. Stir in the cream and season to taste. If you want your soup a little thinner add extra stock. Put the parsley, saved cauliflower, and an optional drizzle of olive oil in bowls and finish with it.

4.6 Herby broccoli & pea soup

(**Prep. time:** 30 min. | **Servings:** 4 | **Difficulty:** easy)

Serving size: 1 cup

Per serving: Kcal 214, Fat 8g, Carbs 19g, Proteins 12g

Ingredients

- 1 tbsp. rapeseed oil
- 1 onion, chopped
- 1 garlic clove, crushed
- Broccoli small florets 400g
- Frozen peas 300g
- Chopped chard 200g
- 1lb. low-salt veg stock
- ½ bunch basil, chopped
- Chopped bunch of dill
- 1 lemon, zested and juiced
- 2 tbsp. toasted pumpkin seeds

Directions

1. Heat up the oil in a large pan. Add the onions and fry until tender and transparent, for 8 minutes. Add the garlic, and simmer for another 1 min. Tip the broccoli, peas, and chard, then spill over the stock & bring to boil, the mixture. Reduce heat for 25 min. to a simmer, cover and serve.

2. Mix in the spices, the lemon zest and juice, then blitz the soup with a stick blender till smooth. Ladle into bowls & serve with the toasted pumpkin seeds sprinkled over the surface.

CHAPTER 5 POULTRY

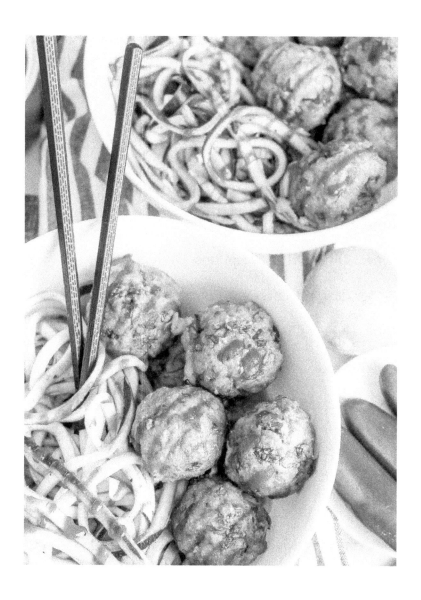

5.1 Zippy Turkey Zoodles

Eating healthy doesn't mean sacrificing flavor—and these spiced-up zoodles prove it. If you don't have a spiralizer, simply slice the zucchini julienne-style

(Prep. time: 45 min. | **Servings:** 4 | **Difficulty:** easy)

Serving size: 1 ¾ cup

Kcal: 332, Fats: 14g, Carbs: 21g, Proteins: 29g

Ingredients

- Olive Oil, 4 Teaspoons, Divided
- Ground Turkey, 1 Pound
- Finely Chopped Onion, 1 Small
- Seeded And Chopped Jalapeno Pepper, 1
- Minced Garlic Cloves, 2
- Ground Cumin, ¾ Teaspoon
- Salt, ½ Teaspoon
- Chili Powder, ¼ Teaspoon
- Red Pepper Crushed Flakes, ¼ Teaspoon
- Pepper, ¼ Teaspoon
- Zucchini, Spiralized, 3 Medium

- Chopped Plum Tomatoes, 4

- 1 cup thawed frozen corn

- Black beans, rinsed and drained

- Optional: fresh cilantro, chopped, and cheddar cheese, shredded

Directions

1. Heat large nonstick frying pan, add 2 tsp. olive oil on medium heat. Stir in onion, garlic, turkey, and jalapeno.

2. Cook until meat has changed color and veggies are soft,

3. Break up turkey into crumbles, after 8-10 minutes, and drain. Mix in the seasonings; remove from heat and keep warm. Clean the pan.

4. In the same frying pan, heat the remaining olive oil stir fry zucchini until crisp and tender over medium heat for about 3-5 minutes.

5. Mix r in corn, beans, tomatoes, and set aside turkey mixture; heat thoroughly. Serve with cheese and cilantro, if desired.

5.2 General Cho's Stew

Asian food is full of flavors .this recipe makes a chili-like soup with the typical flavors of General Cho's chicken. Cooking in a slow cooker makes this recipe super easy, and any type of meat can be used. It tastes great with turkey, leftover pork, or ground meats.

(Prep. time: 2hrs. | **Servings:** 6 | **Difficulty:** easy)

Serving size: 1 cup

Kcal: 222, Fats: 9g, Carbs: 10g, Proteins: 25g

Ingredients

- 1 cup tomato juice

- ½ cup cherry peppers pickled, chopped

- 2 tbsp. soy sauce

- 2 tbsp. hoisin sauce

- 1 tbsp. peanut oil

- 1 to 2 tsp. red pepper flakes, crushed

- 1 lb. cooked chicken, shredded

- 1-½ cups chopped onion

- 1 cup fresh broccoli, chopped

- ¼ cup green onions, chopped

- 1 tsp. toasted sesame seeds

Directions

1. In a 4- or 5-¼ sizeable slow cooker, mix the first six ingredients.

2. Add in chicken, broccoli, and onion. Cover and cook on low for about 2 hours, or until vegetables are soft.

3. Garnish with green onions and toasted sesame seeds to serve.

5.3 Perfect Roast Chicken

A hearty dish that can be enjoyed alone, or with veggies or rice. The leftovers can be used in many recipes given in this book.

(**Prep. time:** 1hr. 45min. | **Servings:** 10 | **Difficulty:** easy)

Serving size: 3 oz. without skin

Kcal: 120, Fats: 21g, Carbs: 0g, Proteins: 16g

Ingredients

- 1 roasting chicken, (4 lb.)

- ½ small granny Smith apple, unpeeled and chopped

- ½ small onion, coarsely chopped

- 4 or 5, skins left on garlic cloves

- 8 sprigs thyme, folded over

- 3 sprigs rosemary, folded over

- Kosher salt to taste

- Black pepper, freshly ground, to taste

- 2 tbsp. olive oil, (divided use)

Directions

1. Heat the oven to 475°F. Wash the chicken thoroughly (inside and out) and pat dry.

2. In a medium bowl, combine the onion, apples, garlic, rosemary, thyme, pepper, salt, and 1tbsp. of olive oil.

3. Fill the chicken cavity with an onion-herb mixture. Use a twine to connect the chicken legs together and attach the wings to the chicken frame.

4. Rub the chicken's exterior with the remaining olive oil on all sides, then brush with extra salt and pepper.

5. Cover the roasting pan with the cooking spray and put the chicken on the breast's side in the pan. 45 minutes of open roasting. Using a roasting rack sprayed with cooking spray, if necessary.

6. Place the chicken on its back and roast for another 30-40 minutes, or until the chicken juices are visible. The legs are supposed to move easily. The temperature inside should reach 180°F, and the skin should be golden colored.

7. Let the chicken off the grill. Let it rest on a loosely covering platter for 20 minutes to let the juices cool down and render carving simpler. Take the twine out before carving. Throw away the filling (used for flavoring only) and skin before eating.

5.4 Baked Turkey with Onions & Leeks

Baking pieces of turkey is one of the easiest ways to put a meal on the table for your family. This mustard-glazed chicken is roasted on a bed of sliced onions, leeks, and garlic that you can serve alongside it.

(**Prep. time**: 1hr. 20 min. | **Servings:** 6 | **Difficulty:** easy)

Serving size: 1 Quesadilla

Kcal: 248, Fats: 12g, Carbs: 7g, Proteins: 25g

Ingredients

- 2 cups onions, thinly sliced

- 1 cup leek, thinly sliced, washed, white and light green part only

- 4 garlic cloves, thinly sliced

- 3 tbsp. extra-virgin olive oil, divided

- 2 tsp. thyme leaves fresh

- ¼ tsp. salt

- 2 ½ -3 lb. turkey pieces, skinless, trimmed, (thighs, drumsticks or breasts)

- ¼ cup Dijon Mustard

- 2 tsp. shallot, minced

- 1 ½ tsp. fresh rosemary chopped

- 1 tsp. soy sauce, reduced-sodium

- ¾ tsp. pepper, freshly ground

Directions

1. Oven heated to 400°F.

2. Toss the leek, onion, garlic, 2 tbsp. of oil, salt, and thyme in a wide bowl till the vegetables are well covered. Place the mixture in a 9-by-13-inch baking dish. Layer the pieces of turkey onto the vegetable and s Bake for about 10 minutes.

3. Whisk the mustard, rosemary, shallots, pepper, and soya sauce in a mixing bowl; stir in the remaining 1 tablespoon of oil gradually.

4. Rub the chicken with the mustard glaze after 10 minutes. Proceed baking until the thermometer placed into the thickest section of the leg or breast part is 165°F, about 30 to 45 minutes longer.

5. Serve the turkey and the vegetables.

5.5 Cheesy Chicken and Broccoli

Have your vegetables enjoyed with this nice Creamy Chicken and Broccoli main course dinner. This nutritious dish is suitable for those with diabetes.

(Prep. time: 20 min. | **Servings:** 6 | **Difficulty:** easy)

Serving size: 4-oz chicken & 3 oz. veggies

Per serving: Kcal: 139, Fats: 4g, Carbs: 1g, Proteins: 23g

Ingredients

- Slivered Almonds, ¼ cup

- 2 (10 oz.) packages frozen Broccoli Pcs. in cheese sauce, (cooked according to package directions)

- 3 cups chicken or turkey breast, cubes, cooked

- ¼ cup pimentos, drained, diced

Directions

1. In a small pan, dry roast almonds over medium heat until they brown.

2. In a large pan, put broccoli & cheese sauce. Mix in chicken and pimentos, turn to a Simmer, stirring continuously until broccoli and chicken mixture are heated.

3. Add water to thin sauce if necessary, garnish with toasted nuts before serving.

CHAPTER 6 FISH AND SEAFOOD

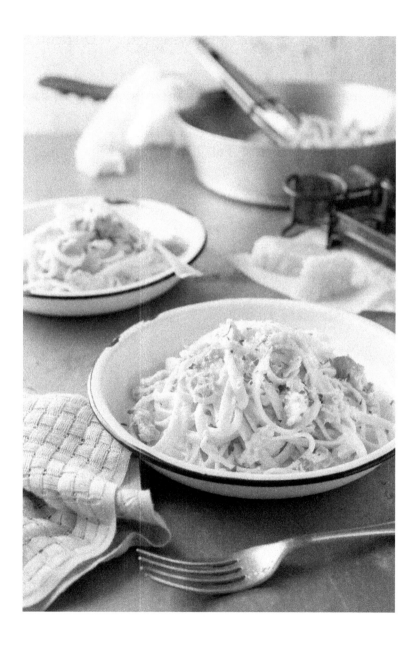

6.1 Salmon Alfredo

(**Prep. time:** 30 min. | **Servings:** 6 | **Difficulty:** medium)

Serving size: 1 cup noodle mixture with $^1/_3$ cup salmon mixture

Per serving: Cal 227, Fat 4.9g, Carbs 23g, Proteins 23.2g

Ingredients

- 3 cups wide noodles

- 3 cups broccoli florets

- 1 ½ cups fat-free milk

- 3 tbsp. all-purpose flour

- 1 tbsp. dried chives

- 2 garlic cloves, minced

- 2 tbsp. grated parmesan cheese

- 1 can salmon, drained, skin & bones removed and broken into chunks

- ½ tsp. shredded lemon peel

- Optional: freshly ground black pepper

Directions

1. Cook the noodles according to the instructions of the box, incorporating broccoli for the last three min. of cooking; drain and warm.

2. Whisk together the milk and flour in a saucepan; add the chives and garlic. Cook and mix until bubbly and thickened, over medium heat. Add the lemon peel as well as salmon. Heat through.

3. Put the noodle mixture on serving dish; top with a spoon of salmon mixture. Sprinkle with Parmesan cheese, and freshly ground black pepper, if necessary.

6.2 One-Pot Pasta with Tuna

(**Prep. time:** 35 min. | **Servings:** 4 | **Difficulty:** easy)

Serving size: 1 cup

Per serving: Cal 382, Fat 15g, Carbs 42.2g, Proteins 21.7g

Ingredients

- 3 ¼ cups water

- 8 oz. whole-wheat spaghetti

- ½ tsp. salt

- ½ cup castelvetrano olives, cut away from the pit

- 2 tsp. fresh lemon zest and juice of ½ lemon

- ½ tsp. ground pepper

- 2 cans unsalted tuna, drained & flaked

- 3 tbsp. chopped fresh dill

- 2 tbsp. extra-virgin olive oil

Directions:

1. In a big, deep skillet, mix the water, spaghetti, olives, lemon juice, lemon zest, salt, and pepper. Bring to a boil, minimize heat to hold a slight simmer, and cook, stirring regularly, 10 to 12 minutes, till most of the water is absorbed & the pasta is tender. Stir in the tuna, dill, and oil but also remove from the heat.

6.3 Greek Tuna Casserole

(**Prep. time:** 1 hr. 15 min. | **Servings:** 6 | **Difficulty:** medium)

Serving size: 1 cup

Per serving: Cal 239, Fat 8.4g, Carbs 23.8g, Proteins 20.2g

Ingredients

- $1/3$ cup dried whole-wheat orzo pasta

- 1 medium eggplant ends trimmed and cut into 1-inch thick slices

- 1 red sweet pepper, stemmed, quartered & seeded

- 2 tbsp. olive oil

- 1 ½ tsp. finely shredded lemon peel

- 2 tbsp. lemon juice

- 1 garlic clove, minced

- 4 tbsp. snipped fresh oregano

- ½ tsp. salt

- ¼ tsp. ground black pepper

- ½ cup panko breadcrumbs

- 3 cans low-sodium tuna, undrained, large pieces broken up,

- ½ cup halved ripe olives

- 1 9-oz. package frozen artichoke hearts, thawed & quartered if needed

- ¼ cup crumbled feta cheese

- Cut 1 lemon into 6 wedges

Directions

1. Preheat the oven to 425°F. Cover with cooking spray a 1 ½-quarter au gratin dish; set aside. Cook pasta according to the instructions on the box. Drain and put aside.

2. Line baking sheet 15x10x1-inch with foil. Coat both sides of every slice of eggplant lightly with cooking spray. Place coated slices of eggplant in prepared baking tray. In a pan of eggplant slices, incorporate the sweet pepper quarters. Uncovered, roast for 15 to 20 min. or until the eggplant starts to brown and the peppers are soft. Remove from the hot oven; let cool. Cut eggplant & pepper into ¾-inch cubes.

3. Reduce the Oven to 350°F.

4. Mix together olive oil, one teaspoon of lemon peel, lemon juice, and garlic in a tiny bowl to make a lemon dressing. Whisk in 3 tablespoons oregano, salt, and black pepper; set it aside. Combine the panko, the remaining 1 tbsp. oregano, as well as the remaining ½ tsp. lemon peel in another small bowl; set aside.

5. Add the cooked orzo, eggplant, sweet pepper, tuna, artichoke heart, olives & feta cheese in a large bowl. Stir in the lemon dressing. Spoon the mixture in prepared baking dish. And cover with foil. Bake in the oven at 350°F for 30–40 min. or until fully heated. Sprinkle panko mixture over the top. Bake for 5 to 8 more min., uncovered, or until the panko mixture becomes golden brown. Using lemon wedges to serve.

6.4 Easy Thai Green Curry with Shrimp

(**Prep. time:** 20 min. | **Servings:** 4 | **Difficulty:** easy)

Serving size: ¼ of the recipe

Per serving: Kcal 228, Fat 9.6g, Carbs 8.7g, Proteins 26.2g

Ingredients

- 1 lb. peeled & cooked shrimps

- 7 oz. snap peas

- 1 can coconut milk

- 3 tbsp. green curry paste

- 1 onion

- 1 garlic clove

- 2 tbsp. fish sauce

- 1 tsp. olive oil

Directions

1. Peel the onion and dice it, then peel the garlic and crush it.

2. Heat a tsp. of olive oil over medium heat in a pan or cast-iron skillet.

3. Stir in the chopped onion & crushed garlic until it is warmed. Sauté once transparent, for a few minutes.

4. Add coconut milk, curry-green paste, & fish sauce. Allow for about 10 minutes to simmer uncovered, or until much of coconut water has evaporated as well as the sauce is nice & creamy.

5. Wash the snap peas, and snap them lengthwise to increase the cooking time.

6. Stir in the coconut curry sauce with the snap peas and simmer for around 1 minute.

7. Add the shrimp and proceed to cook for 30 seconds.

6.5 Grilled Shrimp Skewer with Creamy Chili Sauce

(**Prep. time:** 20 min. | **Servings:** 4 | **Difficulty:** medium)

Serving size: 6-8 shrimps

Per serving: Kcal 134, Fat 2.3g, Carbs 2.4g, Proteins 25.2g

Ingredients

- 1 lb. shrimp
- ½ cup plain Greek yogurt
- ½ tbsp. sambal oiled chili paste
- ½ tbsp. lime juice plus more to topping
- Green onions to topping
- Wooden skewers

Directions

1. Clean & devein the shrimps.

2. Skewer the shrimp, around 5 per skewer.

3. Set shrimp skewers over medium heat on a grill. Grill on either side for 2-3 min., till the shrimps are pink.

4. Remove & top with lime juice and green onions.

For sauce:

5.   Stir Greek yogurt, sambal oiled, and lime juice till well mixed.

CHAPTER 7 VEGETABLES RECIPES

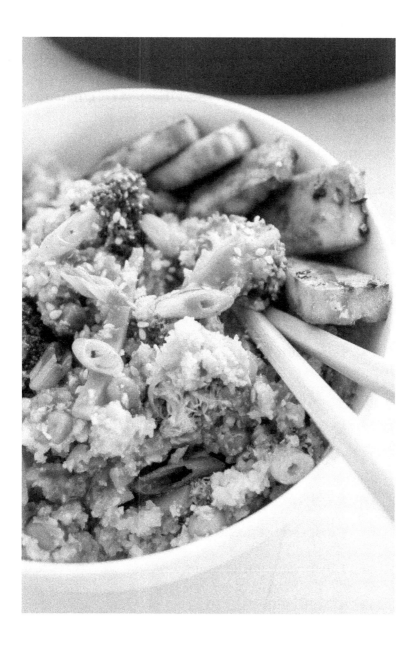

7.1 Stir-Fry Rice Bowls

This meatless edition of Korean Bibimbap is delicious, pleasant and simple to adjust for various spice levels.

(**Prep. time:** 30 min. | **Servings:** 4 | **Difficulty:** medium)

Serving size: ¼ of recipe

Per serving: Kcal: 305, Fats: 11g, Carbs: 40g, Proteins: 12g

Ingredients

- 1 tbsp. canola oil

- 2 medium carrots, julienned

- 1 medium zucchini, julienned

- ½ cup baby Portobello mushrooms, sliced

- 1 cup bean sprouts

- 1 cup baby spinach, fresh

- 1 tbsp. water

- 1 tbsp. soy sauce, reduced-sodium

- 1 tbsp. chili garlic sauce

- 4 large eggs

- 3 cups brown rice hit cooked

- 1 tsp. sesame oil

Directions

1. Heat the canola oil over medium to high heat in a big pan. Put in the carrots, mushrooms, and zucchini; cook and mix for 3–5 minutes or till the carrots are soft and crispy. Add sprouts of bean, spinach, soy sauce, water and sauce of chili; continue cooking until spinach sags. Withdraw from the heat; let it stay warm.

2. Put 2 or 3 inches of water in a big pan with high edges. Let it boil; to sustain a gentle simmer, adjust the heat. Split the cold eggs in a small bowl, one at a time; keep the bowl close to the water surface and drop the egg into the water.

3. Cook 3-5 minutes, without covering, or until whites are fully set, and yolks start thickening but are not stiff. Pick eggs off the water using a large spoon. In plates, serve rice; fill with vegetables. Glaze with the oil of sesame. Put one poached egg with every serving.

7.2 Spinach Quesadillas

My family gave loud cheers and claps to these cheesy quesadillas. Take the spinach off from the fire as soon as it sags so it stays crunchy.

(**Prep. time:** 25 min.| **Servings:** 4| **Difficulty:** medium)

Serving size: 3 wedges

Per serving: Kcal: 281, Fats: 12g, Carbs: 30g, Proteins: 14g

Ingredients

- 3 oz. (about 4 cups) baby spinach, fresh

- 4 chopped green onions

- 1 small chopped tomato

- 2 tbsp. lemon juice

- 1 tsp. ground cumin

- ¼ tsp. garlic powder

- 1 cup Mexican cheese blend/Monterey jack cheese, shredded reduced-fat

- ¼ cup Ricotta cheese, reduced-fat

- 6 (6 inches) flour tortillas

- Sour cream, reduced-fat, your choice

Directions

1. Cook and mix the first six ingredients in a big nonstick pan till the spinach is shriveled. Take off heat; mix in cheeses.

2. With the mixture of spinach, top half of each tortilla, fold another half over the filling. Place on a pan sprayed with cooking spray; cook 1-2 minutes on each side over medium heat until golden brown. Split the quesadillas into half; eat with sour cream if wanted.

Health Tip:

1. Use whole-wheat tortillas and acquire about twice the fiber per portion.

7.3 Quick Mushroom Barley Soup

An easy and nutritious combination, warm and filling!

(Prep. time: 30 min. | **Servings:** 6 | **Difficulty:** easy)

Serving size: 1 cup

Per serving: Kcal: 196, Fats: 7g, Carbs: 27g, Proteins: 8g

Ingredients

- 1 tbsp. olive oil
- 1 cup fresh mushrooms, sliced
- ½ cup chopped carrot
- 1/3 cup chopped onion
- 2 cups water
- ¾ cup barley, quick cooling
- 2 tbsp. all-purpose flour
- 3 cups whole milk
- 1-½ tsp. salt
- ½ tsp. pepper

- Sugar substitute (stevia, Splenda or another one)

Directions

1. Heat oil over low heat in a big saucepan. After adding mushrooms, onion and carrot continue cooking for 5–6 minutes or until soft. Mix in water and barley. Just get it to boil. Lower heat; boil for 12–15 minutes, without covering, or till the barley is soft.

2. Combine the sugar substitute, flour, pepper and salt in a mixing bowl until it becomes smooth; blend well into the broth. Shift to boil, continuously mixing; cook and mix for 1-2 minutes, or until it thickens.

7.4 Hummus & Veggie Wrap-Up

A diner inspired wrap, perfectly flavored for a simple lunch. Can be served with a salad or a dip.

(Prep. time: 15 min. | **Servings:** 1 | **Difficulty:** easy)

Serving size: 1 wrap

Per serving: Kcal: 235, Fats: 8g, Carbs: 32g, Proteins: 7g

Ingredients

- 2 tbsp. hummus
- 1 (8 inches) tortilla, whole wheat
- ¼ cups salad greens, torn mixed
- 2 tbsp. sweet onion, finely chopped
- 2 tbsp. cucumber, thinly sliced
- 2 tbsp. alfalfa sprouts
- 2 tbsp. shredded carrot
- 1 tbsp. balsamic vinaigrette

Directions

1. Layer the hummus on the tortilla.
2. Put on it vegetables, cucumber, onions, carrots and sprouts.
3. Sprinkle the vinaigrette. Fold firmly.

7.5 Zucchini Crust Pizza

The recipe for this special pizza is a dieter's inspiration. It's just perfect for breakfast, lunch or a light dinner. Remove the nutritious zucchini crust from the tray with a metal spatula.

(**Prep. time:** 45 min.| **Servings:** 6| **Difficulty:** medium)

Serving size: 1 slice

Per serving: Kcal: 188, Fats: 10g, Carbs: 12g, Proteins: 14g

Ingredients

- 2 cups squeezed dry, shredded zucchini

- ½ cup egg substitute or 2 large eggs lightly beaten

- ¼ cup all-purpose flour

- ¼ tsp. salt

- 2 cups mozzarella cheese, shredded part-skim, divided

- ½ cup parmesan cheese, divided and grated

- 2 small halved and sliced, tomatoes

- ½ cup red onion, chopped

- ½ cup bell pepper, julienned

- 1 tsp. dried oregano

- ½ tsp. dried basil

- Fresh basil, chopped, your choice

Directions

1. Heat the oven to 450°C. In a big tub, mix the first four ingredients; mix in ½ cup mozzarella and ¼ cup grated parmesan. Move over to a 12-inch. Pizza pan adequately sprayed with a cooking spray; stretched to 11-in. circle.

2. Bake until golden brown for 13-16 minutes. Decrease oven settings to 400°C. Scatter the remaining mozzarella cheese, finish Garnish with tomatoes, ginger, onion, basil and the leftover Parmesan cheese. Bake until the sides are golden brown and the cheese is melted for 10-15 minutes.

3. Garnish with the freshly chopped basil on top, if needed.

CHAPTER 8 PORK LAMB & BEEF

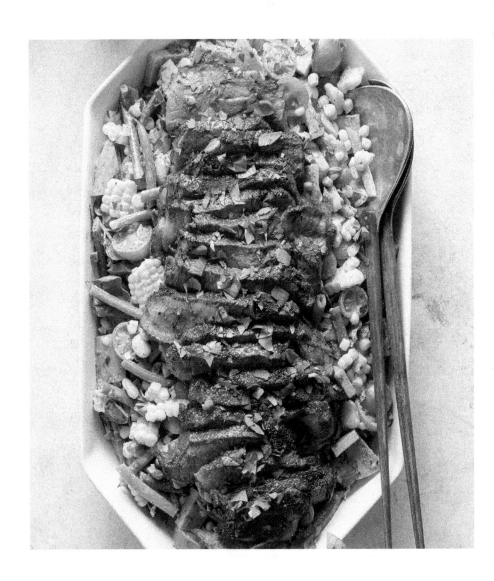

8.1 Succotash Salad with Grilled Sirloin

(Prep. time: 60 min. | **Servings:** 4 | **Difficulty:** medium)

Serving size: 1 ¾ cup salad + 3 oz. steak

Per serving: Kcal 430, Fat 14g, Carbs 46g, Proteins 33g

Ingredients

- 2 cups green beans, cut to pieces of 1-inch and trimmed

- 2 shucked ears corn

- ½ cup Greek yogurt, whole-milk

- 3 tbsp. freshly squeezed lime juice

- Red onion, minced 2 tbsp.

- 2 tbsp. olive oil

- 2 tsp. honey

- 1.5 tsp. garlic, minced

- 1 ¼ tsp. ground pepper

- 1 tsp. salt

- 1 tbsp. chili powder

- 1 tbsp. ground cumin

- 2 tsp. garlic powder

- 1 lb. sweet potatoes, cut to planks of 0.25 inch and peeled

- 1 lb. trimmed top sirloin steak

- 1 cup cherry tomatoes halved

- 1 cup frozen-thawed lima beans

- ¼ cup fresh basil, chopped

- ¼ cup fresh cilantro, chopped

- 1 jalapeño pepper, minced and seeded

Directions

1. Boil ¾ cups of water on medium-high flame in a broad skillet. Add the green beans and cover, decrease heat to medium-low, and steam for about 5 minutes. Drain and transfer into a wide bowl.

2. Fill skillet now empty with water to 2 inches and boil. In the boiling water, add corn and cover, turn the heat off, and steam for about 8 min. Drain corn and put on board; let it cool. Take the kernels from the cobs and move with green beans to the dish.

3. Whisk yogurt, lemon juice, tomato, 1 tablespoon oil, garlic, honey and ¼ teaspoon each salt and pepper.

4. Add cumin powder, chili powder, powdered garlic and the remainder 1 teaspoon ground pepper and ¾ teaspoon of salt in a bowl.

5. Preheat to medium-high grill. Clean grill grate using a wire brush with long handle.

6. Brush the sides of sweet potato with the remainder one tablespoon oil, and season with ½ a mixture of spices. Apply the leftover blend of spices all over the steak. Grill sweet potatoes, 3 to 5 min. per side, until fork-tender. Grill the steak. Place the sweet potatoes onto a cutting board and then let cool. Move the steak to a separate cutting board, and allow 5 minutes to rest.

7. Split the sweet potatoes to 1-inch bits, when cold enough to touch. Slice the steak into 0.5 squares.

8. Add the sweet potatoes and the corn and green beans into the dish. Stir in lima beans, tomatoes, cilantro, basil, and jalapeño; mix with a half cup of the dressing yogurt. Divide salad into 4 dishes. Serve the steak evenly between the plates and drizzle with the yogurt dressing left.

8.2 Stir-Fried Green Beans with Steak & Peanuts

(**Prep. time:** 35 min. | **Servings:** 4 | **Difficulty:** medium)

Serving size: 1 & ¼ cup

Per serving: Cal 362, Fat 26g, Carbs 12g, Proteins 22g

Ingredients

- 1 tbsp. lime juice

- 1 tbsp. fish sauce or reduced-sodium soy sauce

- 3 tbsp. canola oil

- 1 tsp. sugar substitute (Splenda or truvia)

- 12 oz. thinly sliced sirloin steak

- 12 oz. trimmed green beans

- 1 medium red bell pepper, sliced

- 2 garlic cloves, chopped

- ¼ - ½ tsp. red pepper, crushed

- ¼ cup cilantro, chopped fresh

- ¼ cup salted peanuts, chopped

Directions

1. Add lime juice, fish sauce (or soy sauce), 1 tbsp. oil then sugar substitute in a small bowl. Put aside.

2. Heat up 1 tbsp. Oil at medium to high heat in a flat-bottom Carbson-steel wok or large skillet. Add steak; fry, stirring for around 5 minutes, until no longer pink. Move to a bowl. Wipe out the saucepan. Add the remaining 1 tablespoon Oil to the frying pan. Add beans and bell pepper; cook for 7 to 10 minutes , stirring regularly, until the beans are tender-crisp as well as the bell pepper and the beans begin to char. Add the garlic and also the crushed red pepper; cook for 30 seconds to 1 minute longer, stirring, till the garlic is fragrant. Remove from heat. Add reserved combination of lime juice & steak, cilantro, and peanuts. Stir to blend.

8.3 Pressure Cooker "Corned" Beef & Cabbage

(**Prep. time:** 2 hrs. | **Servings:** 8 | **Difficulty:** medium)

Serving size: 3 oz. beef and 1 & $^2/_3$ cups vegetables

Per serving: Cal 295, Fat 10.1g, Carbs 19.2g, Proteins 32g

Ingredients

- 2 ½ lb. trimmed flat-cut beef brisket

- 2 tbsp. ground pickling spice

- 1 tsp. kosher salt

- 2 tbsp. extra-virgin olive oil

- 2 cups low-sodium beef broth

- 1 medium onion, chopped

- 2 lb. halved crosswise carrots

- 1 green cabbage, cut into eight wedges

Directions

1. Mix beef with pickling spice and half teaspoon salt. Heat oil to sauté mode in an electronic pressure cooker. Add the beef & cook, turn once till browned on both sides, a total of around six minutes.

2. Add broth plus onion to the pot. Close & lock your lid. Cook for 40 min., under high intensity. Let all the pressure escape naturally.

3. Press Cancel. Shift the beef to cutting board such that the onion and liquid are left in the pot. Add the carrots, cabbage & the remaining ½ teaspoon salt, with the cooker in Sauce mode. Cook, stirring regularly, for around 20 minutes, till the veggies are soft and the liquid decreases by half.

4. Dice the beef and eat with the veggies and, if necessary, drizzle with the liquid.

8.4 Lamb Chops with Orange Sauce

(**Prep. time:** 20 min. | **Servings:** 4 | **Difficulty:** medium)

Serving size: 2 lamb chops with sauce

Per serving: Cal 250, Fat 10g, Carbs 5g, Proteins 31g

Ingredients

- ½ cup freshly squeezed orange juice

- 2 tbsp. orange zest

- ½ tsp. fried thyme

- ⅛ tsp. ground black pepper

- ½ cup dry white wine

- Nonstick cooking spray

- 8 (about ½-inch thick) lean lamb chops

- 1 cup fresh mushrooms, sliced

Directions

1. Mix the orange juice, orange zest, thyme, & pepper in a small baking dish; stir well.

2. Trim any excess fat from the chops of the lamb and put it in a baking dish. Spoon the mixture of orange juice over the chops; cover, & refrigerate for 3-4 hrs. turning chops periodically.

3. Cover a wide skillet with nonstick spray; position over medium-high flame until hot. Take the chops out from the marinade and conserve the marinade; place them in the skillet. Brown both sides of the chops, remove from the skillet and put on a tray lined with paper towels.

4. Reduce to medium flame, incorporate the mushrooms, & sauté until soft. Add the reserved marinade & wine, and bring to boil.

5. Return the chops of the lamb to the skillet; cover, minimize heat and cook for 10-12 min. or until the sauce has been reduced to around ½ cup. Move the chops of the lamb to a pan, spoon the orange sauce over it and eat.

6. Serve these tasty orange lamb chops with French green beans or baby peas.

8.5 Marinated Leg of Lamb

(**Prep. time:** 40 min.| **Servings:** 16 | **Difficulty:** medium)

Serving size: 3-½, 4 oz.

Per serving: Kcal: 200, Fat: 8g, Carbs: 0g, Proteins:29g

Ingredients

- 3 cups dry red wine
- 1 leg of lamb, boned, butterflied and fat removed
- ¼ cup extra virgin olive oil
- 1 medium onion, sliced
- 1 thinly sliced carrot
- 6 parsley sprigs
- 2 bay leaves, crumbled
- 4 garlic cloves, minced
- ⅛ tsp. freshly ground black pepper
- Fresh parsley sprigs

Directions

1. Combine all ingredients except the parsley sprigs in a large ceramic, glass, or stainless-steel dish (anything but plastic); cover, refrigerate, and allow to marinate for 1–2 days, turning periodically.

2. Drain the lamb after it has been marinated, discard the marinade & pat dry. If needed, season with salt. Put the lamb in a basket with grill. Broil the lamb for 15–20 min. per side, 3 to 4 inches from heat.

3. Place the lamb on a cutting board and then let it cool down slowly. Diagonally carve the lamb; move to a serving platter, garnish it with sprigs of parsley and serve.

4. Serve with sautéed carrots & potatoes cooked in the oven.

CHAPTER 9 DESSERTS

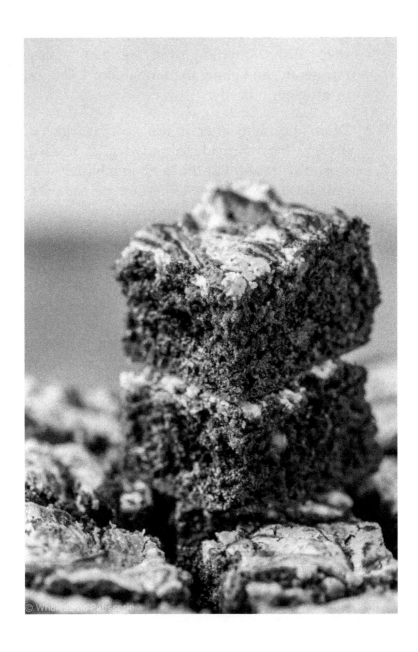

9.1 Peanut Butter Swirl Chocolate Brownies

This diabetic-friendly brownie recipe uses the classic flavor combo of chocolate and peanut butter to yield a tasty cookie that you would want to make over and over again.

(**Prep. time:** 40 min. | **Servings:** 20 | **Difficulty:** hard)

Serving size: 1 brownie

Per serving: Kcal: 151, Fats: 3g, Carbs: 17g, Proteins: 3g

Ingredients

- Non-stick cooking spray
- ¼ cup butter
- ¾ cup sugar substitute (Splenda or truvia)
- ⅓ cup cold water
- 3 lightly beaten eggs
- ¼ cup canola oil
- 1 tsp. vanilla
- 1 ¼ cup tsp. pastry flour, whole-wheat divided
- 1 tsp. baking powder

- ¼ cup peanut butter, creamy

- ½ cup cocoa powder, unsweetened

- ¼ cup small semisweet chocolate pieces

Directions

1. Heat the oven to 350°F. Cover a 9x9x2-inch baking pan with foil, spreading it over the vertices of the pan. Brush foil with non-stick spray, gently. Place aside.

2. Melt butter in a medium saucepan over low heat; take off the heat. Mix in sugar substitute and water. Add in milk, oil, and vanilla until adequately mixed. Place peanut butter in a small bowl; steadily blend in ½ cup of batter until moist. Stir in 1 cup of flour and baking powder until mixed (batter would be thin at this point) place aside. Combine the excess ¼ cup flour in another tub.

3. Shift peanut butter batter over chocolate batter in a saucepan in little piles. Mix batters around, using a small metal spatula. Bake for 20 to 25 minutes or, when pressed gently, the top back and a toothpick inserted near the middle looks dry. Cool down on a wire rack entirely. Round it up into pieces.

Tips

Choose Splenda(R) Sugar Mix for Baking or Sun Crystals(R) instead of granulated sugar, if using a sugar substitute. Check the instructions to use the amount of product that is equal to ¾ cup granulated sugar. Decrease the baking time to 15 to 18 minutes or until the top springs back when pressed gently, and the toothpick put in the middle comes out dry.

9.2 No-Bake Coconut Cream Pie

Are you looking for a delicious dessert abundant in taste but low in Carbs? You're going to enjoy this tropical pie! And it's great for days when you want to keep out of the kitchen and in the sun with no baking needed!

(Prep. time: | Servings: 12 **| Difficulty:** medium)

Serving size: 1 slice

Per serving: Kcal: 118, Fats: 5g, Carbs: 18g, Proteins: 4g

Ingredients

- 2 tbsp. water

- 1 packet (¼ oz.) unflavored gelatin

- 1 can (about 14 oz.) fat-reduced coconut milk

- 1 package (8 oz.) free-fat cream cheese

- 9 packets sugar substitute or equal to 6 tablespoons sugar, divided

- 2 tsp. vanilla

- 1 tsp. coconut extract

- 1 cracker pie crust, reduced-fat graham

- ¼ cup toasted unsweetened flaked coconut

Directions

1. Put water in a relatively small microwave dish. Sprinkle the gelatin over the water; let it rest for 1 minute. Microwave for 20 seconds or before gelatin dissolves entirely.

2. Merge coconut milk, cream cheese, eight sugar substitute packets, vanilla, almond extract, and gelatin mixture in a blender; blend until creamy. Pour into prepared crust; cover and cook for around 4 hours, or until solid.

3. Toast coconut in a small non-stick pan over low heat until golden brown, before eating. Toss coconut with one packet of sugar substitute leftover; spread over pie. Serve ASAP.

9.3 Creamy Strawberry-Banana Tart

What's more delicious than the strawberry and banana mix of iconic flavors? Savor this enjoyable and stylish tart recipe for your taste buds!

(**Prep. time:** 2 ½ hours │ **Servings:** 10 │ **Difficulty:** medium)

Serving size: 1 slice

Per serving: Kcal: 113, Fats: 2g, Carbs: 20g, Proteins: 3g

Ingredients

- 1 package (16 oz.) thawed strawberries, unsweetened and frozen

- Frozen orange juice concentrate, thawed, divided, 2 tablespoons plus 1 ½ teaspoon

- Sugar substitute, ¼ cup (Splenda or truvia)

- 1 envelope (¼ oz.) unflavored gelatin

- 3 beaten egg whites

- 1 package (3 oz.) split, soft ladyfingers

- Water,4 teaspoons

- ½ (8-oz.) container fat whipped topping reduced

- 1 medium banana, sliced and quartered lengthwise

- Optional: 1 tsp. decorative multi-colored sprinkles

Directions

1. In a blender or food processor, put defrosted strawberries and two tablespoons of orange juice concentrate; mix until even.

2. In a medium saucepan, add the sugar substitute and gelatin. Whisk in a mixture of strawberries till well mixed. Cook on medium heat, stirring regularly until they simmer.

3. Mix around half the strawberry mix into thoroughly whisked egg whites. Transfer mixture to the casserole. Cook, stirring continuously, for around 2 minutes or until partially thickened, over medium heat. Never simmer. Pour over into a big bowl. Refrigerate, stirring regularly, for 2 to 2½ hours, or until mixture piles up when spooned.

4. Divide all the ladyfingers in half, lengthwise. Arrange a 9-inch tart pan around the edge with a flexible rim. Place the remaining ladyfingers in the bottom of the saucepan and cut to match. In a shallow cup, mix the remaining 1 ½ teaspoon orange juice concentrate and water. Sprinkle over paned ladyfingers.

5. Fold the whipped topping and banana into a mixture of strawberries; spoon into a ladyfinger crust. Chill for at least 2 hours. If necessary, sprinkle with sprinkles. Cut ten pieces.

9.4 Raspberry Crumble Bars

A dessert waiting to be consumed in your moment of weakness. Can be made ahead and stored

(**Prep. time:** 50min. | **Servings:** 16 | **Difficulty:** medium)

Serving size: 1 slice

Per serving: Kcal: 253, Fats: 24g, Carbs: 8g, Proteins: 4g

Ingredients

Bottom Layer:

- 2 cup almond flour

- 2 cups unsweetened desiccated coconut

- ½ cup coconut Flour

- 4 tbsp. coconut oil, melted

- 6 tbsp. sugar-free syrup/honey/maple syrup

- 2 tbsp. vanilla extract

- ¼ tsp. salt

- 8-10 tbsp. water

Raspberry Chia Jam:

- 3 cup frozen raspberries

- ¼ cup water

- ½ cup chia seeds

- ¼ cup sugar-free syrup/maple syrup /honey

- ¼ cup tsp. vanilla extract

Top Layer:

- 1 cup coconut chips

- 1/3 cup almond flour

- ½ cup unsweetened coconut, desiccated

- 3 tbsp. sugar-free sweet liquid

- 2 tbsp. coconut oil

- ¼ tsp. salt

Directions

1. Heat oven up to 350°F (180°C).

2. Line a square baking tray of 8 inches with parchment paper.

3. Put aside.

Bottom Layer:

1. In a food processor, add the almond meal, coconut flour desiccated coconut, honey,

coconut oil, salt, vanilla, and water (start with 8 tbsp.) until all gets crumbly and the ingredients are combining together. If the mix is too crumbly – add 2 tbsp. of water to come together as a ball when you press in your hands. Always add 2 tbsp. at a time and check the dough. If it holds well, then you have added enough water.

2. Press the batter evenly into the lined baking tray.

3. Flatten the layer using fingers or pressing with a spatula.

4. Prick the base with a fork a few times on few areas to prevent the base from rising when baking.

5. Bake for 15 minutes. Let it cool in the tray thoroughly, then spread the raspberry jam on top.

Raspberry Chia Seed Jam:

1. Prepare the jam, as the bottom layer is in the oven. In a small pan, add all the jam ingredients. Cook the jam on medium-low heat, stirring continuously to avoid any burning. When the raspberry melts totally and thickens, the jam is ready. It will work around 5-6 minutes, not more than that.

2. Set the jam aside and let to cool down fully; it will thicken a little bit more.

3. Spread the jam on the baked layer and return to the oven for another10 minutes to set.

4. Take out from the oven. Put aside, then prepare the final layer.

Top Layer:

1. Put all the top layer ingredients into a big mixing bowl. Using your hand, combine the ingredients together., rub the liquid sweetener and coconut oil onto the dry ingredients to make a crumbly mixture

2. Crumble this mixture on top of the last layer: the chia jam layer, and put the tray back into the oven for another 10 minutes to lightly toast the coconut crumble layer.

3. Cool down for at least 1 hour in the pan. The jam must be at room temperature and set before making slices. Can be stored for up to a week in an airtight container.

9.5 Low Carbs Chocolate mug cake with Coconut Flour

How can a recipe book be complete without a go-to easy dessert as a Choco mug cake, ready in a few minutes to satisfy your sweet tooth?

(**Prep. time:** 6 min. | **Servings:** 1 | **Difficulty:** easy)

Serving size: 1 mug cake

Per serving: Kcal: 167, Fats: 18g, Carbs: 7g, Proteins: 12g

Ingredients

- 1 egg
- 2 tbsp. Erythritol
- 2 tbsp. unsweetened almond milk/milk of your choice
- 1 tbsp. coconut oil/melted butter
- ½ tsp. baking powder, or ¼ tsp. baking soda
- 2 tbsp. almond flour
- 1 tbsp. coconut Flour
- 1 tbsp. unsweetened cocoa powder
- Optional: 1 tbsp. sugar-free chocolate chips

Toppings-optional:

- 1 tsp. peanut butter, to drizzle on top

- 1 tsp. sugar-free dark chocolate

Directions

1. In a small mixing bowl, whisk egg, unsweetened almond milk, erythritol, baking soda, and oil.

2. Mix in coconut flour, almond meal, and unsweetened cocoa powder.

3. Spoon mixture into a mug.

4. Microwave for 1 min increasing by 30 seconds burst if required. It is done when the top is firm and pops out of the mug.

5. Serve immediately. You may drizzle a bit of creamy peanut butter or melted sugar-free dark chocolate on top of the topping.

CONCLUSION

Your children deserve a healthy, simple and fun diet. All the time, it is necessary to have new options of dishes for the children of the house and for those guests that you want to surprise. Just follow this recipe book and dare to give health to your loved ones through meals that will help them with their mental dexterity, integral health and most importantly, you will control the evolution of that Diabetic condition that you are worried about.

Very soon you will begin to notice the substantial changes in the mood of your family environment, the energy in your body, your good digestion and a remarkable weight loss without affecting your sugar level.

Remember that:

1.- This is the beginning of your family's new life.

2.- It is not a vegan / vegetarian diet.

3.- You can transform yours food habits and have fun while you do it.

4.- Grains, vegetables and sauces are your main allies from now on!

CPSIA information can be obtained
at www.ICGtesting.com
Printed in the USA
BVHW041516190321
602997BV00010B/579